Staying Fit: A Comprehensive Guide To Health and Fitness

ABRAHAM ADESEYE

DEDICATION

Dedicated to those who seek to improve their health and fitness, and embrace a lifestyle of wellness and self-care. May this book guide and inspire you on your journey towards a happier, healthier you.

Contents

Welcome to " Staying Fit: A Comprehensive Guide to Health and Fitness." In this book, I will delve into the world of health and fitness, and explore the many benefits that come with living a fit and active lifestyle. Whether you're just starting out on your fitness journey, or you're an experienced fitness enthusiast looking to take your training to the next level, this book has something for everyone.

In today's fast-paced world, it can be easy to neglect our health and fitness, but it's more important than ever to prioritize these aspects of our lives. Regular exercise and a healthy diet can have a profound impact on our physical and mental wellbeing, and they are key to preventing chronic health conditions and improving our quality of life.

In this book, I will cover the basics of health and fitness, and explore the importance of setting achievable goals. I will discuss the role of nutrition in a healthy lifestyle, and provide practical tips and advice on how to make healthy food choices. You will also learn about a range of physical activities and exercises that can help you to achieve your fitness goals, and I will cover the importance of rest and recovery, and how to avoid injury.

Throughout the book, I will share inspiring stories from real people who have transformed their health and fitness through hard work and dedication. Whether you're a busy working parent, a student, or a senior citizen, these stories will show you that it's never too late to start living a healthy and active lifestyle.

In addition to providing practical tips and advice, this book is also designed to be a valuable resource for anyone looking to improve their health and fitness. From learning about the latest fitness trends and exercises, to exploring the benefits of mindfulness and meditation, this book has everything you need to get started on your journey to better health and fitness.

So whether you're just starting out, or you're looking to take your fitness to the next level, this book is here to support you every step of the way. With hard work, dedication, and a commitment to your health and fitness goals, there's no limit to what you can achieve. So let's get started on this exciting journey to a better you, and take the first step towards a healthier, happier, and more fulfilling life.

1 INTRODUCTION TO HEALTH AND FITNESS

Health and fitness are two interrelated concepts that are essential to our overall well-being. Fitness refers to the physical ability to perform tasks and activities, while health is a state of complete physical, mental, and social well-being. The two concepts go hand in hand, and when one is optimized, it leads to an improvement in the other.

In this chapter, I will delve into the basics of health and fitness, exploring the various components that make up a healthy lifestyle. I will also touch on the importance of setting achievable health and fitness goals, and how they can help you maintain a healthy lifestyle in the long term.

The Basics of Health and Fitness

Health and fitness are integral components of overall well-being, and they play a crucial role in supporting both physical and mental health. While the terms are often used interchangeably, they each have their own distinct definitions and significance.

Health refers to the overall state of the body and mind, and it encompasses physical, mental, and emotional well-being. Health is influenced by a range of factors, including genetics, lifestyle choices, and access to healthcare. A healthy lifestyle involves making choices that support overall health, including eating a balanced diet, engaging in regular physical activity, getting adequate sleep, managing stress, and avoiding harmful habits such as smoking and excessive alcohol consumption.

Fitness, on the other hand, refers to the ability of the body to perform physical tasks effectively and efficiently. Fitness can be improved through regular exercise and physical activity, which helps to strengthen the muscles, improve cardiovascular health, and enhance endurance. Physical fitness is important not only for physical health but also for mental well-being, as it can help to reduce stress, improve mood, and boost self-esteem.

In order to achieve and maintain good health and fitness, it is important to adopt a holistic approach that encompasses both physical and mental well-being. This can involve engaging in regular exercise and physical activity, eating a balanced diet, managing stress, and taking care of the mind and body through self-care and mindfulness practices.

Health and fitness are essential components of a happy and fulfilling life, and they play a crucial role in supporting both physical and mental well-being. By making healthy lifestyle choices and engaging in regular physical activity, you can improve your overall health and fitness, and enjoy a happier and more fulfilling life.

The Importance of Setting Achievable Health and Fitness Goals

Setting achievable health and fitness goals is an important step in any fitness journey, and it can be a powerful tool for motivation and progress. Goals give you a clear direction and focus, and they help you to track your progress and celebrate your successes along the way.

Having clear, achievable health and fitness goals can help you to stay motivated and focused, and it can provide a sense of accomplishment and satisfaction as you reach each milestone. It is important to set goals that are specific, measurable, and achievable, and that align with your personal values and priorities.

For example, instead of setting a vague goal of "getting in shape," a more specific and achievable goal might be "to run a 5K race in three months." This type of goal is specific, measurable, and has a clear deadline, which makes it easier to track progress and stay motivated.

In addition to setting specific and achievable goals, it is also important to create a plan for how to achieve them. This may include developing a training plan, tracking your progress, and seeking support from friends and family.

Another important factor in setting achievable health and fitness goals is being realistic and patient with yourself. It is important to remember that progress takes time, and that setbacks and challenges are a normal part of the journey. By focusing on progress, not perfection, and celebrating small victories along the way, you can stay motivated and committed to your goals, even when faced with obstacles.

Setting achievable health and fitness goals is an important aspect of any fitness journey, and it can be a powerful tool for motivation and progress. By setting specific, measurable, and achievable goals, and by creating a plan for how to achieve them, you can stay focused, motivated, and on track towards your health and fitness goals.

Before embarking on a fitness journey, it is crucial to understand your body and its needs. Every person is unique, and each body has its own set of requirements and limitations. In this chapter, I will explore the different body types, how to determine your body type, and how to cater to its specific needs.

I will also discuss the importance of regular medical check-ups and how they can help you stay on top of your health. Whether it's an annual check-up or a visit to a specialist, it's essential to be proactive about your health and stay on top of any potential issues.

The Different Body Types

In the world of health and fitness, it's important to understand that everyone is unique, and this extends to our bodies as well. Different people have different body types, each with its own set of strengths and challenges. Understanding your body type is an important part of creating a personalized fitness and nutrition plan that will help you to achieve your goals.

There are three main body types: ectomorph, mesomorph, and endomorph. Ectomorphs are typically thin and lean, with a light frame and long limbs. They have a fast metabolism, and can find it challenging to gain weight and muscle mass. Mesomorphs are typically athletic and muscular, with a balanced build and a moderate metabolism. They have an easier time gaining muscle mass, but can also put on weight if they are not careful with their diet. Endomorphs have a slower metabolism and a tendency to store fat easily. They may struggle with weight gain, but they also have a natural advantage when it comes to building muscle mass.

To determine your body type, it's helpful to consider your genetic makeup, as well as your current physical characteristics and lifestyle. You can also look at family history, as body type tends to run in families. However, it's important to remember that body type is just one factor in determining your overall health and fitness, and that everyone can benefit from a healthy diet and regular exercise, regardless of their body type.

Once you have a better understanding of your body type, you can tailor your fitness and nutrition plan to meet your specific needs. For example, if you're an ectomorph, you may need to focus on high-calorie, high-protein foods to help you build muscle mass. If you're an endomorph, you may need to focus on portion control and regular exercise to help you maintain a healthy weight. And if you're a mesomorph, you may need to pay extra attention to your diet to avoid putting on unwanted weight, while also engaging in regular strength training to build and maintain muscle mass.

Understanding your body type is an important step in creating a personalized fitness and nutrition plan that will help you to achieve your goals. Whether you're an ectomorph, mesomorph, or endomorph, with the right plan and a commitment to your health and fitness, you can live a happy, healthy, and active life.

The Importance of Regular Medical Check-Ups

Regular medical check-ups are an important part of maintaining good health, regardless of your age, body type, or fitness level. By visiting a healthcare provider on a regular basis, you can stay on top of any potential health issues, and take proactive steps to prevent them from becoming more serious.

One of the key benefits of regular check-ups is early detection. If you have a health issue, such as high blood pressure, high cholesterol, or a chronic condition like diabetes, your healthcare provider can identify it in its early stages and start you on a treatment plan to manage it before it becomes more serious. Early detection also means that you have more options for treatment, and a better chance of making a full recovery.

Regular check-ups also help you to stay on top of preventative measures, such as getting vaccines, screenings, and regular check-ins with your healthcare provider. By staying up to date on recommended screenings and vaccinations, you can reduce your risk of serious health problems, and keep your body in good working order.

In addition to physical health, regular check-ups can also help you to manage your mental health. Your healthcare provider can assess your overall well-being, and provide you with support and resources to help you manage stress, anxiety, or depression. This can include therapy, medication, or a combination of both, depending on your needs and goals.

Finally, regular check-ups can help you to build a relationship with your healthcare provider, which can be especially beneficial in an emergency. If you have a pre-existing health condition, your provider will be more familiar with your health history and can provide more informed care if you need it.

Regular medical check-ups are an important part of maintaining good health and wellness. By visiting your healthcare provider on a regular basis, you can stay on top of any potential health issues, stay up to date on preventative measures, manage your mental health, and build a relationship with your healthcare provider. So, make sure to schedule your next check-up today and take the first step towards better health and wellness!

Nutrition is a crucial aspect of health and fitness, and it plays a vital role in determining how our body performs and how we feel. In this chapter, I will explore the different food groups, how to balance your meals, and the importance of portion control.

I will also discuss the various supplements and vitamins available, and when they are necessary to support a healthy diet. Whether you're trying to lose weight, build muscle, or simply maintain a healthy lifestyle, this chapter will provide you with the information you need to make informed decisions about your diet.

The Different Food Groups

Balancing your meals and paying attention to portion control are key components of a healthy diet. To achieve a balanced diet, you should aim to consume a variety of foods from different food groups, including:

Fruits and vegetables: These are essential sources of vitamins, minerals, and fibre. Aim to eat a variety of different coloured fruits and vegetables to get a range of nutrients.

Grains: Grains provide energy, fibre, and important nutrients. Whole grains are the best option, as they contain more fibre and nutrients than refined grains.

Protein: Protein is important for building and repairing tissues, and for maintaining a healthy immune system. Good sources of protein include lean meats, poultry, fish, beans, and tofu.

Dairy: Dairy provides calcium and other important nutrients, such as vitamin D and potassium. Low-fat or fat-free options are best for maintaining a healthy weight.

Fats: Fats are an important part of a healthy diet, but it is important to choose healthy fats, such as those found in nuts, seeds, and oils, over unhealthy fats, such as those found in processed snacks and baked goods.

To balance your meals, aim to include foods from each of these food groups at each meal. For example, a healthy lunch might include a salad with grilled chicken, a whole grain roll, and a serving of fruit.

Portion control is also an important part of a healthy diet. Portion sizes have increased in recent years, which can lead to overeating and weight gain. To control portions, you can use smaller plates, eat more slowly, and pay attention to hunger and fullness cues. You can also measure out portions of food using measuring cups or a food scale to help you get a better understanding of how much you should be eating.

A balanced diet and portion control are important components of a healthy lifestyle. By eating a variety of foods from different food groups and paying attention to portion size, you can ensure that you are getting the nutrients you need to maintain good health and wellness. So, start by making small changes to your diet today, and work towards a healthier and happier you!

The Various Supplements and Vitamins Available

Supplements and vitamins can be a great way to support a healthy diet and meet your nutrient needs, but it's important to understand that they should not be used as a substitute for a balanced diet. Eating a variety of nutrient-dense foods is the best way to meet your nutritional needs.

Here are some common supplements and vitamins that are often used to support a healthy diet:

Multivitamins: A daily multivitamin can help fill any nutrient gaps in your diet, but it's important to choose a high-quality supplement that is appropriate for your age, sex, and health status.

Vitamin D: Vitamin D is important for bone health, and many people do not get enough from their diet. A vitamin D supplement can be helpful, especially during the winter months when sunlight exposure is limited.

Calcium: Calcium is important for bone health, and many people do not get enough from their diet. A calcium supplement can be helpful, especially for those who do not consume dairy products.

Omega-3 fatty acids: Omega-3 fatty acids are important for heart health, and many people do not get enough from their diet. A fish oil supplement is a common way to get these essential fatty acids.

Probiotics: Probiotics are beneficial bacteria that can help improve gut health. They are commonly found in fermented foods, such as yogurt and kefir, but can also be taken in supplement form.

It's important to talk to your doctor or a registered dietitian before starting any new supplements, as some can interact with medications or have side effects. Your healthcare provider can help you determine if a supplement is necessary for you and help you choose the best option for your needs.

Supplements and vitamins can be a helpful addition to a healthy diet, but they should not be used as a substitute for a balanced diet. Eating a variety of nutrient-dense foods, and talking to your doctor or a registered dietitian about any necessary supplements, is the best way to support your health and wellness.

A healthy diet is the foundation of a healthy lifestyle, and it starts with building a healthy meal plan. In this chapter, I will guide you through the process of creating a nutritious and balanced meal plan that works for you.

I will discuss the importance of eating a variety of foods, including fruits, vegetables, lean proteins, and whole grains. I will also touch on the benefits of cooking at home, and how it can help you make healthier food choices.

Additionally, I will provide you with tips and tricks for eating out and making healthy food choices while on the go. Whether you're busy at work, traveling, or simply don't have time to cook, this chapter will provide you with the information you need to make healthy food choices, no matter where you are.

Creating a Nutritious and Balanced Meal Plan

Creating a nutritious and balanced meal plan is a great way to support your overall health and wellness. A balanced meal should include a variety of food groups, including carbohydrates, proteins, healthy fats, and plenty of fruits and vegetables. Here's a step-by-step guide to creating a nutritious and balanced meal plan:

Determine your daily caloric needs: This can be done using a calorie calculator or by talking to a registered dietitian.

Your daily caloric needs will depend on your age, sex, weight, height, and activity level.

Choose a variety of food groups: Aim to include a variety of food groups in each meal, including whole grains, protein, healthy fats, and plenty of fruits and vegetables.

Incorporate protein: Protein is essential for muscle building and repair, and can help you feel full and satisfied. Good protein sources include lean meats, poultry, fish, beans, and tofu.

Choose healthy carbohydrates: Complex carbohydrates, such as whole grains and starchy vegetables, are a great source of energy and help regulate blood sugar levels.

Add healthy fats: Healthy fats, such as avocados, nuts, and olive oil, are important for heart health and can help you feel full and satisfied.

Eat plenty of fruits and vegetables: Fruits and vegetables are a great source of vitamins, minerals, and fibre, and should make up a large portion of your diet.

Popular meal plans, such as the Mediterranean diet, DASH diet, and the Flexitarian diet, are great examples of how to create a balanced and nutritious meal plan.

The Mediterranean diet is a great example of how to include a variety of food groups in each meal. This diet emphasizes whole grains, fruits and vegetables, healthy fats from sources like olive oil, and lean proteins from sources like fish.

The DASH diet is a diet that was created to lower blood pressure and is focused on reducing salt and sodium intake.

This diet emphasizes whole grains, fruits, vegetables, and lean proteins, and limits the consumption of processed and high-fat foods.

The Flexitarian diet is a plant-based diet that emphasizes plant-based proteins, such as legumes, tofu, and seitan, and allows for the occasional consumption of meat and animal products. This diet is focused on reducing meat consumption and increasing the consumption of plant-based foods.

Creating a nutritious and balanced meal plan is a great way to support your overall health and wellness. By including a variety of food groups, such as whole grains, protein, healthy fats, and plenty of fruits and vegetables, and by following popular examples, such as the Mediterranean diet, DASH diet, and the Flexitarian diet, you can ensure that your meal plan is both balanced and nutritious.

The Benefits of Cooking at Home

Cooking at home has many benefits for your health, wellness, and overall quality of life. Here are some of the key benefits of cooking at home:

Better nutrition: When you cook at home, you have control over the ingredients you use, allowing you to choose healthier options and avoid harmful additives, preservatives, and excess salt and sugar. This can help you improve your overall nutrient intake and maintain a healthy diet.

Increased fruit and vegetable consumption: Cooking at home often involves incorporating more fruits and vegetables into your meals, which can increase your overall nutrient intake and improve your health.

Cost savings: Cooking at home is often more cost-effective than eating out or relying on pre-packaged meals. This can help you save money while also allowing you to make healthier choices.

Better portion control: When you cook at home, you have control over the portion sizes of each meal, which can help you avoid overeating and maintain a healthy weight.

Improved cooking skills: Cooking at home allows you to experiment with new recipes and ingredients, which can help you develop your cooking skills and expand your culinary knowledge.

Quality time with family and friends: Cooking at home can be a fun and social activity, allowing you to spend quality time with family and friends while preparing and sharing meals together.

Increased food safety: When you cook at home, you have control over the preparation and storage of your food, reducing the risk of foodborne illnesses and allowing you to maintain food safety.

Cooking at home has numerous benefits for your health and wellness. By incorporating healthy ingredients, portion control, and food safety practices, cooking at home can help you improve your overall quality of life.

Tips and Tricks for Eating Out

Eating out can be a challenge when trying to maintain a healthy diet, but with a few simple tips and tricks, it's possible to make healthy food choices while on the go. Here are some of the key strategies to keep in mind:

Plan ahead: Research menu options and make a plan for what you'll order before you arrive at the restaurant. This can help you avoid impulse decisions and ensure you make a healthier choice.

Choose wisely: Look for menu items that are grilled, baked, broiled, or steamed, as these are typically healthier options than fried or sautéed dishes. Additionally, opt for dishes with plenty of vegetables, lean proteins, and whole grains.

Control portion sizes: Share an entree with a friend or ask for a to-go box when your meal arrives and immediately divide your meal in half, so you're not tempted to overeat.

Ask for modifications: Don't be afraid to ask for modifications to your meal, such as extra vegetables or a sauce on the side. Restaurants are often happy to accommodate requests to make your meal healthier.

Be mindful of condiments: Condiments, such as salad dressing and sauces, can add a lot of extra calories to your meal. Opt for low-fat or reduced-calorie options, or ask for them on the side so you can control how much you use.

Stay hydrated: Drink plenty of water throughout the meal, as this can help you feel full and avoid overeating.

Look for healthier options on the go: When eating on the go, look for healthier options such as fresh fruit, yogurt, or a salad. Avoid high-calorie, processed foods like pastries, chips, and candy.

By following these tips, you can make healthier food choices while eating out and on the go. With a little planning and mindfulness, you can maintain a healthy diet and enjoy meals out without sacrificing your health.

5 UNDERSTANDING DIFFERENT TYPES OF EXERCISE

Exercise is a crucial aspect of health and fitness, and it plays a vital role in improving physical and mental well-being. In this chapter, I will explore the different types of exercise, including strength training, cardiovascular training, and flexibility training.

I will discuss how to incorporate them into your routine for optimal results. Whether you're looking to build muscle, lose weight, or simply improve your overall fitness, this chapter will provide you with the information you need to make informed decisions about your exercise routine.

The Different Types of Exercise

Exercise is a critical component of a healthy lifestyle, and there are several different types of exercise that can help you achieve your health and fitness goals. Here's a closer look at some of the most important types of exercise:

Strength training: Strength training involves using resistance to build muscle and increase overall strength. This can be done through lifting weights, using resistance bands, or using bodyweight exercises like push-ups and squats. Strength training is important for building muscle, improving bone density, and maintaining overall health as you age.

Cardiovascular training: Cardiovascular training, also known as aerobic exercise, is any activity that increases your heart rate and breathing for an extended period of time. Examples include running, cycling, swimming, and using a cardio machine like a treadmill or stationary bike. Cardiovascular training is important for improving heart health, burning calories, and boosting overall fitness.

Flexibility training: Flexibility training involves stretching and moving your body in ways that increase flexibility and range of motion. This can include yoga, Pilates, and other forms of stretching exercises. Flexibility training is important for reducing the risk of injury, improving posture, and maintaining overall mobility.

It's important to incorporate a variety of different types of exercise into your routine in order to achieve a well-rounded, balanced workout regimen. This can help you avoid injury, improve your overall fitness, and keep your workouts fresh and interesting. Additionally, it's important to remember that different types of exercise will benefit different people in different ways, so it's important to experiment and find what works best for you.

Incorporating Strength, Cardiovascular, and Flexibility Training into Your Routine

Incorporating strength, cardiovascular, and flexibility training into your routine is a key part of achieving optimal health and fitness results. Here are some tips for making sure each type of exercise is well-represented in your workout routine:

Strength Training: Aim to strength train at least two to three times a week, focusing on different muscle groups each time. Start with lighter weights and gradually increase the resistance as your muscles become stronger. Incorporate exercises like squats, deadlifts, and lunges into your routine, along with exercises that target your arms, chest, back, and core.

Cardiovascular Training: Aim to engage in cardiovascular exercise for at least 30 minutes a day, five days a week. This can include activities like running, cycling, swimming, or using a cardio machine. Mix up your routines to avoid boredom and to challenge your body in different ways. For example, try interval training one day and a steady-state cardio session the next.

Flexibility Training: Incorporate flexibility training into your routine at least two to three times a week. Start with a warm-up to prepare your muscles, and then spend 10 to 15 minutes stretching your major muscle groups. Consider incorporating yoga or Pilates into your routine, which can help you improve your flexibility, balance, and posture.

It's important to remember that everyone's fitness goals and needs are different, so what works for one person may not work for another. The key is to listen to your body and make adjustments as needed, whether that means modifying the intensity, duration, or frequency of your workouts. With time and consistency, you'll be able to find the right balance of strength, cardiovascular, and flexibility training to help you achieve your health and fitness goals.

Strength training is a type of exercise that focuses on building muscle and improving overall physical strength. In this chapter, I will guide you through the basics of strength training, including how to perform different exercises, how to choose the right weights, and how to avoid injury.

I will also discuss the benefits of strength training, including increased muscle mass, improved bone density, and reduced risk of injury. Whether you're a beginner or an experienced fitness enthusiast, this chapter will provide you with the information you need to safely and effectively incorporate strength training into your routine.

Building Muscle

Building muscle and improving overall physical strength is a key aspect of a comprehensive fitness routine. Here are some tips for maximizing your results:

Use proper equipment: Make sure you have access to appropriate equipment, such as dumbbells, barbells, and resistance bands. Choose weights that are challenging but manageable, and adjust your weights as needed as your strength improves.

Learn proper form: It's important to learn the correct form for each exercise to avoid injury and get the most out of your workout. Consider working with a personal trainer or using online resources to help you perfect your technique.

Focus on compound exercises: Compound exercises are those that work multiple muscle groups at once. Examples include squats, deadlifts, and bench presses. By focusing on these exercises, you can effectively target multiple muscle groups in a single workout, saving time and maximizing results.

Start with lighter weights: When starting out with strength training, it's important to start with lighter weights and gradually increase resistance as your muscles become stronger. This will help you avoid injury and ensure that you are making steady progress.

Increase resistance gradually: To build muscle, it's important to challenge your muscles with heavier weights over time. Start with lighter weights and gradually increase the resistance as your muscles become stronger. This will help you avoid injury and ensure that you are making steady progress.

Incorporate progressive overload: Progressive overload is a technique where you gradually increase the weight or resistance you're using to challenge your muscles. This can help you see continuous improvements in strength and muscle size.

Don't neglect your diet: Building muscle requires adequate protein, as well as sufficient calories to support muscle growth. Make sure you're eating a balanced diet that includes plenty of lean protein, healthy fats, and complex carbohydrates to fuel your workouts and support muscle growth.

Get adequate rest and recovery: Adequate rest and recovery is crucial for building muscle and improving overall physical strength. Make sure to allow yourself adequate time to rest between workouts, and don't be afraid to take a day off if you're feeling tired or run down.

Avoid overtraining: Overdoing it with strength training can lead to injury and burnout. Make sure to allow yourself adequate time to rest between workouts and to avoid pushing yourself too hard.

Mix up your routine: Finally, it's important to mix up your routine to avoid boredom and to challenge your muscles in different ways. Consider trying new exercises, switching up your workout routines, or incorporating different types of training, such as HIIT or plyometrics.

Remember, building muscle and improving physical strength takes time and consistency, but with the right approach, you can achieve your health and fitness goals and feel stronger and more confident in your body. By incorporating strength training into your fitness routine and following these basics, you can effectively build muscle, improve physical strength, and support your overall health and well-being.

The Benefits of Strength Training

Strength training provides a wide range of benefits for both physical and mental health. Here are some of the key benefits of incorporating strength training into your fitness routine:

Increased muscle mass: Regular strength training can help increase muscle mass, which can boost overall physical strength and improve athletic performance.

Improved bone density: Strength training can help improve bone density, reducing the risk of osteoporosis and other age-related conditions.

Reduced risk of injury: By strengthening muscles and improving flexibility, strength training can help reduce the risk of injury, both in everyday life and during physical activity.

Improved metabolism: Building muscle mass can help boost your metabolism, allowing you to burn more calories even when you're not working out.

Better balance and coordination: Strength training can help improve balance and coordination, reducing the risk of falls and other accidents.

Better posture: Regular strength training can help improve posture by strengthening the muscles that support your spine and core.

Increased self-confidence: Building physical strength through strength training can help boost self-confidence and self-esteem, improving mental health and well-being.

Better sleep: Regular strength training can help improve sleep, reducing the risk of sleep disorders and promoting overall health.

Reduced stress: Engaging in strength training can help reduce stress and anxiety, promoting better mental health and well-being.

By incorporating strength training into your fitness routine, you can enjoy these and many other benefits, helping you achieve optimal physical and mental health and well-being.

Cardiovascular exercise is a type of exercise that helps improve the function of your heart and lungs, and is essential for maintaining good health. In this chapter, I will discuss the various types of cardiovascular exercise, including running, cycling, and swimming.

I will explore the benefits of cardiovascular exercise, including improved heart health, increased endurance, and weight loss. Additionally, I will provide tips and tricks for incorporating cardiovascular exercise into your routine, and how to make it enjoyable and sustainable in the long term.

The Various Types of Cardiovascular Exercise

Cardiovascular exercise is a type of physical activity that involves repetitive, rhythmic movement of large muscle groups, such as the legs, arms, and torso. This type of exercise is designed to raise the heart rate and increase blood flow, improving cardiovascular health and endurance. Here are some of the most popular types of cardiovascular exercise:

Running: Running is one of the most popular forms of cardiovascular exercise, and it's easy to see why. It's an accessible and inexpensive way to get your heart rate up, and it's a great way to improve cardiovascular health and endurance.

Cycling: Cycling is another popular form of cardiovascular exercise, and it's a great way to improve cardiovascular health, build endurance, and strengthen the legs and core.

Swimming: Swimming is a low-impact form of cardiovascular exercise, making it a great choice for those who are recovering from injury or who want to avoid high-impact exercise. Swimming is also a full-body workout that can help improve cardiovascular health, build endurance, and strengthen the muscles.

Elliptical training: Elliptical training is a low-impact form of cardiovascular exercise that simulates running or walking but without the impact on the joints. This type of exercise is great for improving cardiovascular health, building endurance, and strengthening the legs, arms, and core.

Rowing: Rowing is a full-body workout that combines cardiovascular exercise with strength training, making it a great choice for those who want to improve both cardiovascular health and overall physical strength.

Jump rope: Jump rope is a simple but effective form of cardiovascular exercise that can be done almost anywhere. It's a great way to improve cardiovascular health, build endurance, and strengthen the legs, arms, and core.

These are just a few of the many types of cardiovascular exercise available. By incorporating different types of cardiovascular exercise into your fitness routine, you can improve your cardiovascular health, build endurance, and enjoy a range of physical and mental health benefits.

The Benefits of Cardiovascular Exercise

Cardiovascular exercise is an essential component of a healthy lifestyle, providing numerous physical and mental health benefits. Here are some of the most significant benefits of incorporating cardiovascular exercise into your routine:

Improved heart health: Regular cardiovascular exercise can help improve heart health by strengthening the heart muscle, increasing blood flow, and reducing the risk of heart disease.

Increased endurance: Cardiovascular exercise can help improve endurance by strengthening the heart and lungs, allowing you to work out for longer periods of time and with less fatigue.

Weight loss: Cardiovascular exercise is an effective way to burn calories and lose weight, making it a great choice for those who are trying to shed excess pounds.

Improved mental health: Cardiovascular exercise has been shown to have a positive impact on mental health, reducing stress, anxiety, and depression, and improving overall mood.

Better sleep: Regular cardiovascular exercise has been shown to improve sleep quality, allowing you to get a better night's rest and wake up feeling refreshed and energized.

Improved joint health: Cardiovascular exercise can help improve joint health by reducing joint stiffness and pain, and reducing the risk of injury.

Reduced risk of chronic disease: Regular cardiovascular exercise has been shown to reduce the risk of chronic diseases such as stroke, diabetes, and certain types of cancer.

Improved immune function: Cardiovascular exercise has been shown to improve immune function, helping you fight off infections and illnesses more effectively.

Incorporating cardiovascular exercise into your routine is a simple and effective way to improve your overall health and wellness, and to enjoy a range of physical and mental health benefits. So whether you prefer running, cycling, swimming, or another type of cardiovascular exercise, make sure to include it as part of your regular fitness routine.

Tips and Tricks for Incorporating Cardiovascular Exercise into Your Routine

Incorporating cardiovascular exercise into your routine is a great way to improve your overall health and wellness, but it can be challenging to stick with it if it doesn't feel enjoyable or sustainable. Here are some tips and tricks for making cardiovascular exercise a regular part of your routine:

Find an activity you enjoy: Choose a type of cardiovascular exercise that you enjoy, such as running, cycling, swimming, or dancing. This will make it easier to stick with it in the long term.

Set achievable goals: Start with small, achievable goals, such as walking for 10 minutes a day, and gradually increase the duration and intensity of your workouts as you get stronger.

Make it a social activity: Invite a friend to join you for your workouts, or join a class or club where you can exercise with others. This can make it more enjoyable and help you stay motivated.

Vary your routine: Mix up your routine by trying different types of cardiovascular exercise, such as running one day and cycling the next. This will keep things interesting and help you avoid boredom.

Use technology to track your progress: Use a fitness app or tracker to monitor your progress, set goals, and track your progress. This can help you stay motivated and on track.

Incorporate other forms of physical activity: Incorporate other forms of physical activity, such as yoga or stretching, into your routine to complement your cardiovascular exercise and keep your body balanced.

Listen to music or audio books: Use music or audio books to help pass the time and make your workouts more enjoyable.

Make it part of your routine: Set a regular time for your cardiovascular exercise and make it a non-negotiable part of your daily routine, just like brushing your teeth or taking a shower.

By incorporating these tips and tricks into your routine, you can make cardiovascular exercise a sustainable and enjoyable part of your life. So whether you're just starting out or looking to take your workouts to the next level, make sure to incorporate cardiovascular exercise into your routine and enjoy all of its many benefits.

Flexibility training is a type of exercise that focuses on improving your range of motion and reducing the risk of injury. In this chapter, I will discuss the different types of flexibility training, including stretching and yoga.

I will explore the benefits of flexibility training, including improved posture, reduced muscle stiffness, and reduced risk of injury. Additionally, I will provide tips and tricks for incorporating flexibility training into your routine, and how to make it a regular part of your fitness journey.

The Different Types of Flexibility Training

Flexibility training is an important aspect of a well-rounded fitness routine, as it helps to improve the overall function and mobility of the body. There are various forms of flexibility training, including stretching and yoga, and each offers unique benefits.

Stretching is a simple and accessible form of flexibility training that can be done anywhere, at any time. Stretching involves holding a position for a certain amount of time that stretches a specific muscle group. Regular stretching can help to improve flexibility, posture, and reduce the risk of injury. For those who are just starting out with flexibility training, stretching is a great place to start. There are many online resources and videos available that can help you learn different stretches and how to do them properly.

Yoga is a more comprehensive form of flexibility training that involves not just stretching, but also mindfulness, breathing exercises, and meditation. There are various styles of yoga, ranging from slow-paced, gentle yoga to fast-paced, power yoga. Some of the more popular styles include Hatha yoga, Vinyasa yoga, and Bikram yoga. Yoga is great for increasing flexibility, strength, balance, and mental focus, and it has been found to have numerous physical and mental health benefits. For example, regular yoga practice has been shown to reduce stress, improve sleep, and lower blood pressure. Additionally, yoga can be a fun and social activity, as there are many studios and classes available where you can practice with others.

When starting with flexibility training, it is important to listen to your body and not push too hard too soon. Gradually incorporating stretching and yoga into your fitness routine is the best approach. You may also find it helpful to work with a qualified instructor or teacher, who can help you learn proper techniques and avoid injury.

Incorporating flexibility training into your routine can help you achieve a better overall balance of strength, cardiovascular health, and flexibility. By taking the time to stretch and do yoga, you can improve your overall physical and mental well-being, and reduce the risk of injury. So make sure to make flexibility training a priority in your fitness routine, and you will be on your way to a healthier, happier you!

The Benefits of Flexibility Training

Flexibility training has numerous benefits that contribute to a healthy and well-rounded fitness routine. The following are some of the key benefits:

Improved Range of Motion: Flexibility training helps increase the range of motion in your joints, which can help reduce the risk of injury during physical activity. This is especially important for individuals who engage in activities that require a lot of movement, such as athletes or those who engage in manual labour.

Reduced Muscle Soreness: Regular stretching can help reduce muscle soreness and tightness after intense physical activity. This is because stretching helps to improve circulation and increase blood flow to the affected areas.

Improved Posture: Flexibility training, especially yoga, can help improve posture. Poor posture can lead to chronic pain and discomfort in the neck, back, and shoulders. By improving flexibility in the muscles and joints, you can help alleviate these issues and maintain good posture throughout the day.

Reduced Risk of Injury: When your muscles are tight, you are more susceptible to injury, particularly during physical activity. Flexibility training helps to keep your muscles relaxed and supple, reducing the risk of strains and sprains.

Reduced Stress and Improved Mood: Flexibility training, particularly yoga, has been shown to help reduce stress and anxiety. This is because the stretching and breathing exercises involved in these activities can help to calm the mind and reduce tension in the body.

Improved Balance: Improving flexibility in the muscles and joints can help improve overall balance, which is especially important as we age. This can reduce the risk of falls and other accidents, and help maintain independence and mobility.

Incorporating flexibility training into your routine can be a great way to complement your other exercise activities and help improve your overall health and wellness. Whether you choose stretching, yoga, or another form of flexibility training, it's important to be consistent and make it a part of your regular routine for maximum benefits.

Tips and Tricks for Incorporating Flexibility Training into Your Routine

Flexibility training is an essential aspect of a well-rounded fitness routine, and it can provide numerous benefits to help you feel more relaxed, flexible, and mobile. Incorporating flexibility training into your routine can be challenging, but with a few tips and tricks, you can make it a regular part of your fitness journey.

Here are some suggestions for incorporating flexibility training into your routine:

Make it a part of your warm-up: Before starting your strength or cardiovascular training, spend 5-10 minutes performing light stretching exercises to warm up your muscles and increase your range of motion. This will help prevent injury and prepare your body for more intense activity.

Dedicate specific time to flexibility training: Set aside time each week specifically for flexibility training, and make it a non-negotiable part of your routine. This could be in the form of a yoga class, stretching routine, or simple stretching exercises at home.

Get creative: There are many different forms of flexibility training, so get creative and find what works best for you. Try different yoga poses, stretching techniques, or even acrobatics to keep things interesting and fun.

Make it enjoyable: The key to making flexibility training a regular part of your routine is to enjoy it. Find a form of flexibility training that you enjoy, and make it a fun and enjoyable part of your fitness journey.

Listen to your body: It's important to listen to your body when performing flexibility training. Avoid pushing yourself too hard and only perform exercises that feel comfortable and safe for you.

By incorporating these tips and tricks into your routine, you can make flexibility training a regular and enjoyable part of your fitness journey. Whether you're a beginner or an experienced fitness enthusiast, the benefits of flexibility training cannot be ignored, and incorporating it into your routine will help you feel more relaxed, flexible, and mobile.

Maintaining a healthy lifestyle is a long-term commitment, and it can be challenging to stay motivated, especially when you reach a plateau. In this chapter, I will discuss the various challenges that people face when trying to maintain a healthy lifestyle, and how to overcome them.

I will explore the importance of tracking your progress, and celebrating your successes. I will also provide tips and tricks for staying motivated, including finding an accountability partner, trying new activities, and setting achievable rewards.

The Various Challenges That People Face When Trying To Maintain a Healthy Lifestyle

Maintaining a healthy lifestyle can be a challenge for many people due to a variety of reasons. One of the most common challenges is a lack of time. With busy schedules, it can be difficult to find time for exercise and meal planning, let alone cooking nutritious meals. Another challenge is a lack of motivation. Sticking to a fitness routine and a healthy diet can be difficult if you don't have the right mindset or support system.

Another challenge is financial constraints. Healthy food options can often be more expensive, and gym memberships or personal training sessions can add up quickly. This can make it difficult for some people to access the resources they need to maintain a healthy lifestyle.

Social and environmental factors also play a role in hindering healthy lifestyle choices. For example, unhealthy food options are often more readily available, and peer pressure can make it difficult to stick to a healthy diet. Moreover, a sedentary lifestyle can be difficult to avoid if you have a desk job or spend a lot of time in front of a screen.

Finally, many people face physical or medical limitations that make it difficult for them to maintain a healthy lifestyle. For example, people with joint pain or arthritis may struggle with certain forms of exercise, while those with food allergies or intolerances may face limitations when it comes to meal planning.

These challenges can make it difficult to maintain a healthy lifestyle, but they are not insurmountable. With the right mindset and support, it is possible to overcome these barriers and achieve your health and fitness goals.

How to Overcome the Challenges

Maintaining a healthy lifestyle can be challenging, but with the right mindset and approach, it is possible to overcome these obstacles. Here are some tips for overcoming the common challenges of maintaining a healthy lifestyle:

Lack of Motivation: It's normal to lose motivation from time to time, but it's important to find ways to stay motivated. Try setting achievable goals, enlisting the help of a friend, or seeking out a support group. Celebrate your progress, no matter how small, and remember why you started your journey.

Lack of Time: Busy schedules can make it difficult to find time for exercise and healthy eating. Try to prioritize physical activity and healthy eating by scheduling it in your daily routine. Incorporate physical activity into your daily routine, like taking the stairs instead of the elevator, or doing a quick workout at home.

Lack of Money: Healthy eating and physical activity can be expensive, but there are ways to save money. Try grocery shopping for in-season produce, meal prepping, and cooking at home. Look for free or low-cost physical activity options, like walking, hiking, or yoga in the park.

Emotional Eating: Emotional eating can be a major challenge for many people. To overcome this, try to identify the triggers that cause you to eat emotionally, and find alternative ways to cope with stress or emotions, like exercise, meditation, or talking to a friend.

Inconsistency: Consistency is key when it comes to maintaining a healthy lifestyle. Try to make healthy choices a habit by incorporating them into your daily routine. Make a plan, and stick to it, even on weekends or when you're traveling.

Remember, maintaining a healthy lifestyle is a journey, and it's important to be kind and patient with yourself. Don't get discouraged by setbacks, instead, learn from them and continue to make progress towards your goals.

The Importance of Tracking Your Progress

Tracking your progress is crucial in maintaining a healthy lifestyle. It helps you see how far you've come, where you need to improve, and keeps you motivated to keep going. By keeping track of your progress, you can see what works for you and what doesn't, allowing you to adjust your plan accordingly. This leads to better results and greater satisfaction with your progress. There are several ways to track your progress, including:

Keeping a journal: Write down your goals, what you eat, and your workout routine. This helps you see what you're doing right and where you can improve.

Using a fitness tracker: Wearable fitness trackers and smartphone apps can help you monitor your activity levels, heart rate, and more.

Measuring yourself: Use a measuring tape to track your body measurements, such as your waist, hips, and thigh circumference. This helps you see the changes in your body composition over time.

Taking progress photos: Take a photo of yourself every few weeks to see how your body is changing.

By tracking your progress, you can make adjustments to your diet and exercise routine as needed, and stay on track towards your health and fitness goals. And, when you see how far you've come, it gives you the motivation and confidence to keep going.

Celebrating Your Successes

Celebrating your successes is an important part of maintaining a healthy lifestyle and reaching your goals. Achieving your health and fitness goals can take time, effort, and dedication, so it's important to take a step back and appreciate your progress along the way. Celebrating your successes can help you feel more motivated and confident in your journey. Here are some tips for celebrating your successes:

Set achievable milestones: Rather than focusing solely on your ultimate goal, break it down into smaller, achievable milestones. This way, you can celebrate your progress along the way and feel a sense of accomplishment.

Treat yourself: After reaching a milestone, treat yourself to something you enjoy. This could be anything from a massage to a special meal. The key is to reward yourself in a way that supports your overall health and fitness goals.

Reflect on your progress: Take some time to reflect on how far you have come. Write down your thoughts, feelings, and experiences and how you have changed since starting your health and fitness journey. This can help you see just how far you have come and how much you have accomplished.

Share your successes with others: Share your achievements with friends and family. Talking about your successes can help you stay accountable, and it can also help you spread positivity and inspiration to those around you.

Celebrating your successes can help keep you motivated and on track. It's a way to acknowledge the hard work you have put in, and it can also help keep you focused on your long-term goals.

Tips and Tricks for Staying Motivated

Staying motivated is key to achieving and maintaining your health and fitness goals. Here are some tips and tricks that can help you stay on track:

Find an accountability partner: Having someone who can hold you accountable can be a great motivator. You can share your goals, progress, and challenges with each other and offer support and encouragement along the way.

Try new activities: If you're feeling bored or unmotivated, trying something new can reignite your excitement for fitness. Try a new workout class, go for a hike, or try a new sport. Mixing things up can help you avoid burnout and keep things interesting.

Set achievable rewards: Reward yourself for meeting your goals. For example, treat yourself to a massage after hitting your fitness milestones, or buy a new workout outfit after reaching a certain weight loss goal. Celebrating your successes can help you stay motivated and focused.

Find a workout buddy: Working out with a friend can make exercise more fun and help you stay motivated. You can encourage each other and hold each other accountable, and it can also help you stay committed to your routine.

Set realistic and achievable goals: Setting achievable goals can help you stay motivated and focused on what you want to achieve. Start with small, achievable goals and then build up as you progress.

Keep track of your progress: Keeping track of your progress, whether it's in a journal, a fitness app, or through tracking your measurements, can help you see your progress and stay motivated.

Take breaks: Taking breaks from your routine can help you avoid burnout and stay motivated. Plan a vacation, take a day off, or try something new to give your mind and body a break.

Remember, it's important to stay positive and focused on your goals, and to celebrate your successes along the way. With dedication and motivation, you can achieve your health and fitness goals and maintain a healthy, active lifestyle.

Injuries and health concerns can be a roadblock in your fitness journey, but they don't have to be. In this chapter, I will discuss the importance of taking care of your body, and how to deal with injuries and health concerns.

I will explore the benefits of working with a professional, such as a doctor, physical therapist, or personal trainer, and how they can help you get back on track. Additionally, I will provide tips and tricks for avoiding injury, including proper form, rest and recovery, and listening to your body.

The Importance of Taking Care of Your Body

Taking care of your body is an important aspect of leading a healthy and fulfilling life. Whether it be through eating well, exercising regularly, or getting enough sleep, taking care of your body is essential for maintaining good health and well-being.

One of the key ways to take care of your body is through proper nutrition. This means eating a balanced diet that is rich in essential vitamins and minerals, and avoiding processed and junk foods that can harm your health. It also means being mindful of portion control and eating regular, balanced meals throughout the day.

Exercise is another important aspect of taking care of your body. Regular exercise helps to keep your heart healthy, improves your stamina and endurance, and strengthens your muscles. Whether it be through strength training, cardiovascular exercise, or flexibility training, it is important to find an exercise routine that works for you and makes you feel good.

In addition to exercise, it is also important to get enough sleep and manage stress. Sleep plays a vital role in physical and mental recovery, and helps to keep your body functioning at its best. Stress, on the other hand, can have negative effects on your health, so it is important to find ways to manage it, such as through relaxation techniques or engaging in stress-relieving activities.

Ultimately, taking care of your body is about making healthy choices on a daily basis and forming habits that promote overall well-being. Whether it be through eating well, exercising regularly, or managing stress, it is important to prioritize your health and treat your body with the care it deserves.

How to Deal with Injuries and Health Concerns

It's essential to address any health concerns and injuries promptly and efficiently to ensure that your fitness journey is not derailed. Here are a few tips for dealing with injuries and health concerns:

Seek medical attention: If you experience any significant pain or discomfort, it's always best to seek medical attention. A doctor or physical therapist can diagnose the issue and provide you with a personalized treatment plan.

Rest and recovery: It's essential to give your body enough time to heal, and avoid putting unnecessary stress on the injured area. This could mean taking a break from physical activity or modifying your routine to avoid putting stress on the affected area.

Physical therapy: Physical therapy can be extremely beneficial in helping you recover from an injury. A physical therapist can work with you to develop exercises to help improve strength, range of motion, and flexibility in the affected area.

Prevention: To reduce the risk of injury, it's important to follow proper form and technique when exercising, warm up adequately before working out, and gradually increase intensity and duration.

Balance your workout: Make sure you're not overdoing it in one area, like strength training, and neglecting other areas, like flexibility training. A balanced workout routine will help reduce the risk of injury and promote overall health and wellness.

Remember, it's crucial to listen to your body and make adjustments as needed. Don't push yourself too hard and always prioritize your health and well-being.

The Benefits of Working with a Professional

Working with a professional can provide numerous benefits for your health and fitness journey. By working with a doctor, physical therapist, or personal trainer, you can receive personalized attention and guidance to help you achieve your goals. Here are a few ways that these professionals can help you get back on track:

Medical Expertise: Doctors are medical experts and can help you address any health concerns you may have. They can perform regular check-ups and help diagnose any medical issues that may be impacting your fitness goals.

Injury Prevention and Treatment: Physical therapists are experts in musculoskeletal injury prevention and treatment. They can help you recover from an injury and get back on track with your fitness routine. They can also show you exercises to help prevent future injuries.

Personalized Workouts: Personal trainers are experts in creating personalized workout plans for their clients. They can help you choose the right exercises to target your specific goals, and make adjustments to your routine as you progress. Personal trainers can also provide motivation and accountability, helping you stay on track and reach your goals.

Proper Technique: Working with a professional can also ensure that you are performing exercises with proper technique. This is important for avoiding injury and maximizing the benefits of your workout.

Working with a professional can provide numerous benefits for your health and fitness journey. By receiving personalized attention and guidance, you can achieve your goals and get back on track with your routine.

Tips and Tricks for Avoiding Injury

In order to avoid injury while exercising, it is important to focus on proper form and technique. This means making sure you are performing each exercise correctly and not straining or overusing any particular muscle group.

It is also important to listen to your body, so if you feel any discomfort or pain, you should stop and rest.

Additionally, it's crucial to incorporate rest and recovery into your routine, as this will give your body time to heal and prevent future injuries.

Stretching before and after your workout can also help to improve flexibility and reduce the risk of injury.

Another key component is to start slowly and gradually increase intensity, as jumping into a high-intensity workout too quickly can put a lot of strain on your body and increase the risk of injury.

Furthermore, it's helpful to seek advice from a professional, such as a doctor, physical therapist, or personal trainer, who can guide you on proper form and technique, help you identify any underlying health issues, and create a safe and effective workout plan tailored to your needs.

Fitness doesn't have to be a chore, and it's essential to make it fun and sustainable in the long term. In this chapter, I will discuss the various ways to make fitness enjoyable, including trying new activities, working out with friends, and setting achievable goals.

I will also explore the benefits of incorporating variety into your routine, and how it can help you stay motivated and avoid boredom. Whether you're a beginner or an experienced fitness enthusiast, this chapter will provide you with the information you need to make fitness a fun and sustainable part of your life.

The Various Ways to Make Fitness Enjoyable

Making fitness enjoyable can be a key factor in helping you maintain a healthy and active lifestyle. Here are some ways to make fitness more enjoyable:

Trying new activities: Experiment with different forms of exercise such as dancing, hiking, or rock climbing. This will help you avoid boredom and keep you motivated.

Working out with friends: Exercise with a partner or join a group fitness class. Having a workout buddy can provide accountability, motivation and make the experience more fun.

Setting achievable goals: Setting achievable goals and tracking your progress can provide a sense of accomplishment and help you stay motivated. Choose goals that are realistic and specific to your needs and abilities.

Music: Create a playlist of your favourite music to listen to while you work out. The right music can help you stay focused and motivated.

Variety: Mix up your routine to include different types of exercise and activities. This will help keep you from getting bored and challenge your body in different ways.

Reward yourself: Celebrate your successes along the way by rewarding yourself for reaching your goals. Treat yourself to a massage, a movie or a special meal.

By making fitness enjoyable, you are more likely to stick with it and reach your health and fitness goals. Incorporating fun and creativity into your workout routine can help make exercise a part of your daily routine.

The Benefits of Incorporating Variety into Your Routine

Incorporating variety into your fitness routine can provide numerous benefits that can help you achieve your health and fitness goals. Firstly, it can help you avoid boredom, which is one of the biggest reasons people tend to lose motivation and give up on their fitness journey. By trying new activities and exercises, you can keep your mind engaged and excited about your workouts, which can in turn help you stick to your routine.

Secondly, incorporating variety into your routine can help you target different muscle groups and improve your overall fitness. For example, alternating between strength training and cardiovascular exercise can help you build muscle and increase endurance at the same time. Similarly, incorporating different types of flexibility training, such as yoga and stretching, can help you improve your balance, posture, and flexibility in a more comprehensive manner.

Thirdly, trying different activities can also help you discover new passions and interests. For example, you may try a new type of dance class and find that you love it, which can then become a new hobby and a source of ongoing exercise.

Finally, incorporating variety into your routine can also help you avoid overuse injuries. By switching between different activities, you give your muscles and joints a chance to rest and recover, reducing the risk of injury.

Incorporating variety into your fitness routine can help you stay motivated, improve your overall fitness, discover new passions, and avoid injury. So, consider trying new activities and incorporating variety into your routine for a well-rounded and enjoyable fitness journey.

12 THE BENEFITS OF MINDFULNESS AND MEDITATION

Mindfulness and meditation are important components of overall health and well-being, and they can have a significant impact on your physical and mental health. In this chapter, I will discuss the various benefits of mindfulness and meditation, including reduced stress, improved focus, and increased self-awareness.

I will explore the different types of mindfulness and meditation practices, including mindfulness-based stress reduction (MBSR), yoga, and breathing exercises. Additionally, I will provide tips and tricks for incorporating mindfulness and meditation into your routine, and how to make it a regular part of your wellness journey.

The Various Benefits of Mindfulness and Meditation

Mindfulness and meditation are practices that have been gaining popularity in recent years, and for good reason. There are numerous benefits associated with incorporating these techniques into your daily routine, including:

Reduced stress: Meditation has been shown to help lower cortisol levels, which is the hormone associated with stress. This reduction in stress can help improve mental and physical well-being, reducing the risk of conditions such as anxiety and depression.

Improved focus: Mindfulness helps you to focus on the present moment, rather than dwelling on the past or worrying about the future. This increased focus can improve productivity, memory, and decision-making abilities.

Increased self-awareness: Meditation can help you become more aware of your thoughts, feelings, and physical sensations, allowing you to understand yourself better and make positive changes to your life.

Improved sleep: Research has shown that mindfulness and meditation practices can help improve sleep quality, leading to better rest and reduced feelings of fatigue.

Improved physical health: Mindfulness and meditation have been linked to lower blood pressure, reduced inflammation, and improved immune system function.

Incorporating mindfulness and meditation into your daily routine can be as simple as taking a few minutes each day to focus on your breath, or participating in guided meditations or yoga classes. It's important to find a practice that works best for you and to be patient as you develop your mindfulness skills. With time and dedication, you'll experience the numerous benefits of mindfulness and meditation for yourself.

The Different Types of Mindfulness and Meditation Practices

Mindfulness and meditation are ancient practices that have been used for centuries to improve mental and emotional well-being. In recent years, they have gained widespread popularity as a tool for reducing stress and improving mental health. There are many different types of mindfulness and meditation practices to choose from, each offering its own unique benefits. Here are a few popular options:

Mindfulness-based stress reduction (MBSR) - This is a well-established program that has been used for decades to help people reduce stress and improve their overall well-being. MBSR combines mindfulness meditation with gentle yoga and body scans to help you become more aware of your thoughts, feelings, and bodily sensations.

Yoga - Yoga is a physical and mental practice that involves holding poses, breathing exercises, and meditation. It has been shown to help reduce stress, improve focus and flexibility, and increase self-awareness.

Breathing exercises - Simple breathing exercises can be a powerful tool for reducing stress and improving mental clarity. Examples include alternate nostril breathing, 4-7-8 breathing, and box breathing.

Regardless of which type of mindfulness or meditation practice you choose, it's important to be patient and persistent. It can take time to see the benefits of these practices, but with regular practice, you will likely experience a greater sense of calm, clarity, and focus in your life.

Tips and Tricks for Incorporating Mindfulness and Meditation into Your Routine

Incorporating mindfulness and meditation into your daily routine can provide numerous mental and physical benefits. Here are some tips and tricks to help make it a regular part of your wellness journey:

Start Small: You don't have to set aside hours each day to practice mindfulness and meditation. Start with just a few minutes each day and gradually increase the time as you get comfortable.

Find the Right Time: Determine the best time of day for you to practice mindfulness and meditation. Some people find it easier to practice in the morning, while others prefer to do it at night before bed.

Use Guided Meditations: Guided meditations can be helpful in the beginning, as they provide structure and guidance. There are many apps, podcasts, and videos available that offer guided meditations.

Find a Quiet Place: Find a quiet place where you can focus on your breath and quiet your mind. If you're just starting out, it may be helpful to use earplugs or noise-cancelling headphones to reduce distractions.

Make it a Habit: Make mindfulness and meditation a daily habit by setting aside a specific time each day to practice. You can also set reminders or use an app to help keep you accountable.

Experiment: Experiment with different types of mindfulness and meditation practices to find what works best for you. Some people prefer mindfulness-based stress reduction (MBSR), while others prefer yoga or breathing exercises.

Be Patient: Mindfulness and meditation take time and practice to see results. Be patient with yourself and trust the process. Remember, it's about the journey, not just the destination.

By incorporating mindfulness and meditation into your daily routine, you'll begin to experience the many benefits, including reduced stress, improved focus, and increased self-awareness.

13 THE IMPORTANCE OF SLEEP FOR HEALTH AND FITNESS

Sleep is an essential component of overall health and fitness, and it plays a vital role in supporting physical and mental well-being. In this chapter, I will discuss the importance of sleep, and how it affects our overall health and fitness.

I will explore the various factors that impact sleep quality, including stress, diet, and technology, and how to improve sleep habits. Additionally, I will provide tips and tricks for getting a good night's sleep, including establishing a bedtime routine, creating a relaxing sleep environment, and limiting caffeine and alcohol consumption.

The Importance of Sleep

Sleep plays a crucial role in our overall health and fitness. It is the time when our bodies repair and restore themselves, and lack of adequate sleep can have negative impacts on our physical and mental well-being. Here are some of the ways in which sleep affects our health and fitness:

Physical health: Lack of sleep can lead to a weakened immune system, increased risk of obesity, and cardiovascular disease. Adequate sleep is necessary for physical repair and restoration, allowing our bodies to recover from physical activity and maintain optimal health.

Mental health: Sleep is essential for maintaining mental clarity and reducing stress and anxiety. Insufficient sleep can lead to irritability, depression, and decreased focus.

Athletic performance: Sleep plays a critical role in athletic performance by enabling our bodies to recover from physical activity and preparing us for the next workout. Poor sleep quality and lack of adequate sleep can lead to decreased energy levels, impaired reaction times, and decreased endurance.

Hormonal balance: Sleep is necessary for maintaining hormonal balance, which affects our metabolism and energy levels. Lack of sleep can disrupt the balance of hormones such as cortisol, insulin, and leptin, leading to weight gain and decreased metabolism.

In order to get the best results from our fitness routines and maintain optimal health, it's important to prioritize sleep and aim for 7-9 hours of quality sleep each night. This means creating a relaxing sleep environment, avoiding screens before bed, and limiting caffeine and alcohol consumption. Additionally, practicing mindfulness and relaxation techniques, such as meditation and deep breathing, can help improve the quality of your sleep and promote overall wellness.

The Various Factors that Impact Sleep Quality

Sleep is essential to our overall health and well-being, as it allows the body to repair and regenerate itself, and supports cognitive function, mood, and energy levels. The quality of sleep we get can be impacted by a range of factors, including stress, diet, and technology. Here are some tips and tricks to improve your sleep habits:

Reduce stress: Stress can make it difficult to fall asleep and stay asleep, so it's important to find ways to reduce stress in your life. This could involve practicing mindfulness or meditation, engaging in physical activity, or finding healthy coping mechanisms.

Watch your diet: Eating too close to bedtime or consuming caffeine, alcohol, or high-fat foods can interfere with sleep. Aim to eat your last meal several hours before bedtime, and choose foods that are high in complex carbohydrates, like whole grains and fruits.

Limit technology use: The blue light emitted by screens, including smartphones, laptops, and televisions, can suppress the production of the sleep hormone melatonin, making it harder to fall asleep. Try to avoid screens for at least an hour before bedtime, or consider using blue light blocking technology.

Establish a bedtime routine: Having a consistent bedtime routine can help signal to your body that it's time to wind down and prepare for sleep. This could include activities like reading, stretching, or taking a warm bath.

Make your sleep environment comfortable: Your sleep environment should be cool, quiet, and dark to promote optimal sleep. Consider using blackout curtains, a white noise machine, or earplugs to minimize distractions.

Set a sleep schedule: Try to go to bed and wake up at the same time every day, even on weekends, to help regulate your internal sleep-wake cycle.

Get physical activity: Regular physical activity can improve the quality of your sleep, but be mindful of the timing. Avoid strenuous exercise close to bedtime, as it can make it harder to fall asleep.

By making these changes, you can improve the quality of your sleep, which in turn will support your overall health and fitness.

Tips and Tricks for Getting a Good Night's Sleep

Establishing a good sleep routine and getting quality sleep is important for overall health and well-being. Here are some tips and tricks to help you get a good night's sleep:

Establish a bedtime routine: Create a routine that you follow every night before going to bed. This could include reading a book, taking a warm bath, or practicing relaxation techniques. Having a consistent routine will signal to your body that it's time to wind down and prepare for sleep.

Create a relaxing sleep environment: Your sleeping environment can have a big impact on the quality of your sleep. Make sure your bedroom is cool, dark, and quiet, and invest in a comfortable mattress and pillows.

Limit caffeine and alcohol consumption: Caffeine and alcohol can both interfere with your sleep. Try to avoid consuming these substances for several hours before bedtime.

Exercise regularly: Regular physical activity can help you fall asleep faster and stay asleep longer. However, it's important to avoid working out within a few hours of bedtime, as exercise can be stimulating and make it difficult to fall asleep.

Limit screen time: The blue light emitted by electronic devices can interfere with your body's production of melatonin, a hormone that helps regulate sleep. Try to avoid using electronic devices for at least an hour before bedtime.

Reduce stress: Stress can keep you up at night and interfere with your sleep quality. Try to reduce stress through activities such as yoga, meditation, or deep breathing.

Keep a sleep diary: Tracking your sleep patterns and habits can help you identify what's working and what's not. You can use a sleep diary to keep track of when you go to bed, when you wake up, and any disruptions during the night.

By incorporating these tips into your routine, you can help ensure that you get a good night's sleep and maintain overall health and wellness.

Maintaining a healthy lifestyle is a long-term commitment, and it requires a sustainable approach. In this chapter, I will discuss the importance of building a sustainable lifestyle for health and fitness, and how to make it a part of your daily routine.

I will explore the various components of a sustainable lifestyle, including a healthy diet, regular exercise, mindfulness, and self-care. Additionally, I will provide tips and tricks for building healthy habits, and how to make them a part of your daily routine.

The Importance of Building a Sustainable Lifestyle for Health and Fitness

Building a sustainable lifestyle for health and fitness is essential for long-term success and well-being. Making healthy choices and being active regularly are the building blocks of a healthy lifestyle, but they can be challenging to maintain in the face of everyday life. Here are some tips and tricks to help you make your health and fitness routine a sustainable part of your daily life:

Start Small: Starting small and gradually increasing the difficulty level is one of the best ways to make fitness a part of your routine. Start with a few simple exercises and add new challenges as you progress.

Set Realistic Goals: Setting achievable and realistic goals is key to making health and fitness a sustainable part of your life. Set small, incremental goals that are within your reach and focus on reaching one goal at a time.

Incorporate Variety: Incorporating variety into your fitness routine is a great way to keep things interesting and prevent boredom. Try new activities, exercises, and workout routines to challenge your body and keep things fresh.

Make it a Habit: Make fitness and healthy eating habits a part of your daily routine. Set aside a specific time each day for exercise, and try to make healthy eating a priority.

Find a Support System: Having a supportive community can help you stay motivated and accountable. Join a gym, workout with friends, or find an accountability partner to help you stay on track.

Reward Yourself: Celebrate your successes and reward yourself for your hard work. Whether it's treating yourself to a massage or buying a new workout outfit, find ways to acknowledge and celebrate your progress.

Be Mindful: Mindfulness and meditation can help reduce stress and improve focus, which is essential for maintaining a healthy lifestyle. Incorporate mindfulness and meditation into your daily routine to help you stay relaxed and focused.

Get Enough Sleep: Sleep is essential for overall health and fitness. Make sure to get enough sleep each night and prioritize rest and recovery in your daily routine.

By following these tips, you can build a sustainable lifestyle for health and fitness that will help you achieve your goals and feel your best. Remember to be patient, stay consistent, and enjoy the journey!

The Various Components of a Sustainable Lifestyle

A sustainable lifestyle for health and fitness involves creating habits and routines that support long-term physical and mental well-being. In addition to a healthy diet, regular exercise, and mindfulness, self-care is an important component of a sustainable lifestyle. Self-care includes activities such as getting enough sleep, managing stress, and taking time for yourself to recharge and relax.

Another important component of a sustainable lifestyle is finding balance. This means avoiding extremes and finding a way to maintain healthy habits while still enjoying life and having fun. For example, indulging in treats every once in a while is fine as long as it is balanced with healthy meals and regular physical activity.

It is also important to be realistic and set achievable goals. Creating too many drastic changes all at once can be overwhelming and lead to burnout. Gradual, consistent changes are more likely to stick and become a permanent part of your lifestyle.

Finally, accountability is key. Having a support system, whether it be friends, family, or a coach, can help you stay on track and maintain motivation. You can also consider tracking your progress and celebrating your successes along the way.

By incorporating these components into your daily routine, you can build a sustainable lifestyle for health and fitness that supports both your physical and mental well-being.

Tips and Tricks for Building Healthy Habits

including setting achievable goals, tracking progress, seeking support from friends and family, and making small, incremental changes to your lifestyle. Building healthy habits is a gradual process and requires patience, determination, and discipline.

Here are some additional tips for building healthy habits:

Start Small: Making big changes to your lifestyle can be overwhelming, so start with small, achievable steps. For example, if you want to eat healthier, start by swapping out sugary drinks for water, or eating a piece of fruit for dessert.

Be Consistent: Consistency is key when it comes to building healthy habits. Establishing a routine and sticking to it will help you establish healthy habits over time.

Celebrate Your Successes: Celebrating small victories along the way will help keep you motivated and on track. Whether it's hitting a fitness milestone, or eating a healthy meal, acknowledge and celebrate your progress.

Create a Support System: Having a support system can make all the difference when it comes to building healthy habits. Surround yourself with people who encourage and motivate you, and seek their support when you need it.

Get Plenty of Sleep: Sleep is an essential component of a healthy lifestyle. Make sure to get enough sleep each night to help you stay focused and motivated throughout the day.

Make it Fun: Incorporating fun and joy into your healthy habits can help make them more sustainable in the long-term. Find activities that you enjoy, such as hiking, dancing, or swimming, and incorporate them into your routine.

Stay Positive: Maintaining a positive attitude is critical to building healthy habits. Stay focused on your goals and the benefits you will reap from making changes to your lifestyle.

Building healthy habits takes time and effort, but it's worth it in the end. With patience, determination, and the right approach, you can create a sustainable lifestyle that promotes health, happiness, and well-being.

Your journey to a healthy and fit lifestyle is an ongoing process, and it's important to celebrate your successes along the way. In this final chapter, I will discuss the importance of celebrating your successes.

I will explore the various ways to celebrate your successes, including setting achievable goals, tracking your progress, and rewarding yourself for your hard work. Additionally, I will provide tips and tricks for staying motivated and committed to your health and fitness journey, and how to make it a lifelong pursuit.

The Importance of Celebrating Your Successes

Celebrating your successes is an essential part of maintaining a healthy lifestyle. It's not only important for staying motivated, but it also helps you recognize your progress and the hard work you've put into achieving your goals. Celebrating your successes provides a much-needed break from the day-to-day grind, and gives you a chance to enjoy the fruits of your labour.

Some tips for celebrating your successes include:

Recognizing your accomplishments: Take time to acknowledge your achievements and reflect on the hard work you've put in. This can help you appreciate your progress and give you a sense of pride in what you've accomplished.

Celebrating with friends and family: Sharing your successes with loved ones can be a great way to bond and make memories. Whether it's a simple celebration or a grand celebration, having others to share in your joy can be incredibly rewarding.

Treating yourself: Treating yourself to something special can be a great way to celebrate your success. It could be something as simple as buying yourself a special treat or taking a relaxing spa day.

Journaling your success: Writing down your successes and accomplishments can be a great way to reflect on your progress. You can look back on your successes and remember the hard work and dedication that went into achieving them.

Track your progress: Keeping track of your progress, either through a journal or an app, is a great way to celebrate your successes. Seeing your progress over time can be a huge motivation boost.

Setting new goals: Celebrating your successes can also be a great time to set new goals and continue on your journey towards a healthy lifestyle. Use your successes as motivation to continue striving towards a better version of yourself.

Try something new: Celebrating your successes by trying something new, such as a new workout class or sport, can be a fun and exciting way to challenge yourself and continue to grow and improve.

Incorporating celebration into your routine can help you stay motivated and on track towards a healthy lifestyle. Remember to take time to celebrate your successes, no matter how small they may seem. Recognizing your accomplishments and taking time to celebrate them can make all the difference in your journey towards a healthier you.

Remember, it's important to celebrate your successes in a way that aligns with your overall health and fitness goals. By taking the time to acknowledge your achievements, you can stay motivated and continue on your journey towards better health and fitness.

Tips and Tricks for Staying Motivated

Surround yourself with supportive people: Surrounding yourself with friends, family, or a workout partner who encourage and motivate you can be a powerful tool for staying motivated. Having someone to share your journey with can also help keep you accountable and provide a sense of community.

Find what works for you: Everyone has different motivators, so it's important to find what works best for you. This could be setting personal challenges, competing against others, or simply finding an activity that you enjoy. Experiment with different forms of exercise and activities until you find what you love and stick with it.

Set achievable goals: Setting achievable, short-term goals can help you stay motivated as you work towards your long-term health and fitness goals. These goals can range from small accomplishments, such as trying a new workout, to larger milestones, such as training for a race or reaching a specific body weight.

Track your progress: Keeping track of your progress, whether it's through a journal, a fitness app, or simply by taking progress photos, can help you see the results of your hard work. This can provide motivation to continue your journey and make any necessary adjustments along the way.

Make it a part of your routine: Incorporating health and fitness into your daily routine can make it a habit and reduce the likelihood of falling off the bandwagon. This could mean setting aside a specific time each day for exercise or preparing healthy meals in advance.

Reward yourself: Celebrating your successes and rewarding yourself for your hard work can be a great motivator. This can be as simple as treating yourself to a massage after a tough workout or buying yourself a new outfit when you reach a specific weight loss goal.

Embrace setbacks: No one is perfect, and setbacks are a normal part of any journey. The important thing is to not give up and to use setbacks as an opportunity to learn and grow. Keep in mind that setbacks are just temporary and can be overcome with hard work and determination.

Stay positive: Maintaining a positive outlook can make a big difference in staying motivated. Surround yourself with positive people and try to focus on the benefits of your journey, rather than the difficulties. Remember that health and fitness is a lifelong pursuit, and taking it one step at a time can lead to lasting results.

In conclusion, health and fitness are essential components of a happy and fulfilling life, and this book provides a comprehensive guide to help you on your journey. Whether you're a beginner or an experienced fitness enthusiast, this book will provide you with the information you need to make informed decisions about your health and fitness, and how to make it a sustainable part of your life.

www.ingramcontent.com/pod-product-compliance
Lightning Source LLC
Chambersburg PA
CBHW051648250726
48653CB00007B/2550